Lyme Disease

A major goal of this book is to offer safe natural treatment solutions to the chronically ill Lyme disease patient and explain the important relationship between correct nutrition and good health. Holistic therapy focuses on the prevention of new symptoms, improving existing symptoms with natural substances and to strengthen the patient's immune system with specific nutrients or herbs.

This book is not intended to replace the services of a licensed physician. Any application of the recommendations set forth in the following pages is at the reader's discretion and sole risk. All life-threatening situations must be treated by the patient's physician.

First printing 2003
Cover design by Hannelore Helbing-Sheafe, Ph.D.

To order additional copies, please contact us.
BookSurge, LLC
www.booksurge.com
1-866-308-6235
orders@booksurge.com

Lyme Disease Alternative Medicine can help

Discussion of
Holistic Therapy Options
for the Prevention and Treatment
of Lyme Disease

Hannelore Helbing-Sheafe, Ph.D.

Huckleberry Hill Press
1547-101st. Ave. S.W.
Olympia, WA 98512-1054

2003

Lyme Disease

Table of content

To my daughters Susanne, Karen
and Christa

Foreword

"Lyme Disease - Holistic Therapy Options" provides valuable information about holistic therapy options for patients afflicted with chronic Lyme disease. The purpose of this book is to provide information about specific natural substances, which can be used to manage the symptoms of Lyme disease; it is not intended to influence the reader's decision, whether to seek only medical care, to seek both medical and holistic counsel, or to consider using only natural and safe remedies in non-crisis situations. Rather, it is suggested to give the holistic point of view careful thought by reading the information presented in this book. Only then can a decision be made based on knowledge and facts. Throughout the ages certain herbs and other natural substances have been used with great success to treat a variety of disease processes. Information about such substances as safe and natural treatment options. will be discussed in this book Orthodox medicine has been unsuccessful in curing patients of Lyme disease. The often complex symptoms are commonly treated with a variety of drugs, which may produce serious side effects. If specific nutrient substances or herbs with well-proven effectiveness could be used instead and not having to worry about side effects, would it not be wise to give these a try? In addition, correct nutrition has always been and always will be the foundation for good health. Lyme disease patients are encouraged to carefully study all available resources on how to properly nourish themselves and use this knowledge to strengthen their bodies against disease.

Hopefully, the information presented in this book will encourage the reader to include alternative therapy in the management of Lyme disease.

Chapter I
What is Lyme disease?

Lyme disease is a bacterial disease, caused by the bite of a "tick" infected with the bacteria known as "Borrelia burgdorferi". The tick, both in the larvae or in the adult stage, transmits the bacteria to humans by attaching itself to any exposed skin area and feeds on its victim. The bacteria then enter the blood, spinal fluid and skin. Not all ticks carry the spirochete bacteria. At this time, all states in the U.S. have reported Lyme disease. Large areas of Europe as well as Australia also are affected. An 8/20/96 announcement by the Lyme board, America Online, states: "Lyme disease is now the second fastest spreading infectious disease in the U.S.A. right behind A.I.D.S". And reports in 2002 describe Lyme disease as a world-wide epidemic. Another publication on Lyme disease reports that scientists have recently discovered other spirochetes, which they believe are capable of causing Lyme disease, or "Lyme-like illness". Other recent articles speak about new outbreaks of tick-borne disease in the U.S.A. These appear to be caused by the same ticks which cause Lyme disease and doctors are instructed to watch for "Erlichiosis" (which evidently responds well to "Doxycycline") and "Babesiosis" (for which no treatment was mentioned). "Erlichiosis" (HGE) causes instant, rather strong symptoms such as nausea, headaches and much fever.

Major areas of tick infestations have been found in California, Oregon, Washington, Nevada and Utah, the upper portions of Wisconsin as well as in the states of Minnesota, Maryland, Massachusetts, Missouri and Texas. However, while these main areas may be the focus of recent studies, tick transmitted disease now shows up just about everywhere in the United States. According to a 1994 publication by the Public Health Department, State of Washington, tick-transmitted disease occurs in most countries of the world. And now that we know more about it, we are able to identify the symptoms, while in years past people became ill and no one knew what was wrong with them.

Lyme disease is not contagious but should be reported to the patient's local health department, so records can be kept and presented to the U.S. Department of Health. Only in the last ten-fifteen years has enough information emerged about how widespread and serious this problem really is.

Identifying different Ticks

Ixodes dammini, called "Deer tick", is found especially in the Eastern part of America. Ixodes dammini is divided into three species: Hermsii, turcicatea and parkeri.

Ixodes pacificus, known as the Western black-legged tick, is found primarily in the Pacific Northwest.

Ixodes angustus is also found in the State of Washington. It is one of the ticks causing Lyme disease.

Lone star tick spirochetes have been found in the state of Missouri. Spirochetes found in this kind of tick cause a "Lyme like illness" and are responsible for a great number of cases in Midwestern states.

According to Dr. Paul Catts, Washington State University, Dept. of Entomology Tick Research, *"Ixodes angustus"* is not usually recognized as a carrier of (infected with) the Borrelia burgdorferi bacteria. The author was infected by an *"Ixodes angustus"* tick late 1994 and the specimen was sent to and identified by Dr. Catts. At that time, Dr. Catts did not expect *"Ixodes angustus"* to carry the bacteria and was amazed, when Public Health Lab in vitro testing produced a "positive" reading. Since all symptoms of an acute infection were also present, there was no doubt that *"Ixodes angustus"* can transmit the "Borrelia burgdorferi" bacteria; Dr. Catts believed this was the first case in Thurston County in the state of Washington.

Where are ticks found?

Ticks are found on shrubs, bushes, in grass and other vegetation. A tick might be brushed off vegetation and then attaches itself to clothing or to unprotected skin areas. *"Ixodes dammini"*, also called "Deer tick", is found in any area, where deer are found, while *"Ixodes angustus"* is more commonly found in the bedding (nests) of chipmunks, wild rabbits and prairie dogs. Cats and dogs can bring ticks into the house. Lizards and goats also may be carriers. In the Eastern states the white-tailed field mouse is known as a carrier.

Human housing built in forests or cleared areas will be affected by ticks. Actually any garden can be home to the tick population. Please, see the chapter "How to landscape for tick protection".

Taking preventive measures

Before going outdoors: Wear trousers, place socks over trouser hems to prevent ticks from gaining entry. Wear a long-sleeved shirt or jacket to protect the arms and upper body. After being outdoors: Clothing and all exposed body parts should be checked for any black specks. Especially the neck, face and head and any exposed body parts should be checked after each outing.

Larvae and infant ticks hang on for feeding and remain, while adult ticks feed and then drop off. And that is the reason, why many people never know that they were bitten by a tick, until characteristic symptoms appear. A physician, questioning the patient about recent outdoor activities, can usually determine that the patient may have been exposed to ticks. The author found a fully engorged *"Ixodes angustus"* tick on her abdomen, transmitted by her dog which hunted chipmunks and rabbits all the time and obviously brought the tick into the home. The bacteria are transmitted to the human body by the tick penetrating the skin and feeding on its host. The reader is advised to call the local County Extension Office and ask for any additional literature. This information should be kept on file for future reference, because ticks are on the march. They are indeed "the new kid on the block".

What happens after the tick bite?

Just how someone reacts to a tick bite depends on that person's general health. If general health is good and the immune system is strong, then the symptoms may not be severe. However, when the infected person already has a disease or a weakened immune system, then the reaction can become quite severe.

There are two basic immediate reactions. There may be local reddening and swelling, or a rash develops as a direct reaction to the bite. The bite site may develop a characteristic large red ring (bulls eye) surrounding the bite area. Fever, chills, vomiting and nausea can occur.

Should a physician be consulted right away?

The answer is yes! If the patient knows or suspects that a tick bite has occurred, he/she should seek immediate medical care, and if possible deliver the tick to the doctor's office. The tick can be carefully removed by using tweezers and very gently pulling straight back. Getting the tick out with the head intact is especially important in order to avoid localized irritation from the bite itself. A special removal kit is available from "Forestry Suppliers, Inc.". Phone: 1-800-752-8460. This kit includes a chemical, which is applied to the feeding tick and causes it to withdraw from its human or animal host. The kit also includes a pair of special removal tweezers and a magnifying lens, so a correct identification can be made. Pharmacies might also have such kits available.

If the tick has engorged itself infection with the spirochete bacteria has already taken place. An engorged tick looks like a plump little tube. It should be removed and saved in a closed container. It is not only important to seek immediate medical treatment but also to have the tick identified as a possible carrier of Borrelia burgendorfi. Treatment with antibiotics must be begun at once. If medical treatment is not immediately available begin treatment with "colloidal silver" at once. Colloidal silver is a highly effective natural and safe antibiotic available in health food stores in liquid form and can easily be stored in a small container and carried during outings.

- Save the tick
- Contact your physician and inform him that you have been bitten by a tick and ask him to immediately have your blood tested and to initiate antibiotic treatment.
- Not every tick carries the spirochete. Yet, it is important in each case to seek a positive identification and to immediately begin preventive treatment just in case.

A new vaccine LYMErix can help to prevent Lyme disease. More information can be found at the AOL WebMD website.

Lyme disease is difficult to diagnose

Lyme disease mimics many different diseases and especially in the beginning produces influenza-like symptoms and fever. A large percentage of individuals bitten by a tick never get the "tell-tale rash". And not every patient responds to the usual medical antibiotic treatment and the disease can and often does become a chronic and constantly relapsing infection.

Incubation period

First symptoms appear within two weeks, but the average is seven days. And, because the patient does not always feel ill right away, and as stated before, it is especially important, to immediately begin antibiotic treatment to prevent the spirochetes from penetrating body cells.

Chapter II
There are three distinctive symptom phases

Phase One - Immediate Reaction

Common symptoms most patients experience:
- Small raised bumps (rash) may cover the entire torso, but fade away after several weeks
- Low-grade temperature
- Some develop a sudden high fever (105 degrees)
- Pulse and rate of respiration increase
- Extreme weakness
- Cough
- Diarrhea
- Eye pain
- Chest pain
- Painful joints
- Muscular pains like rheumatism
- Enlargement of the liver is possible
- Lymph nodes can become involved
- Lymph swelling, especially near the tick bite

- Chills
- Nausea
- Vomiting
- Moderate to severe headache
- Fatigue
- Mental dullness
- Flu-like symptoms
- A red discolored spot (macula) or red pimple (papule) appears at the bite site followed by a particular rash, called Erythema Migrans (EM).
- Within 14 days this rash can expand to twelve inches. The center may clear, so the surrounding tissue takes on a ring-like appearance (bulls eye)
- There may be several rings within the outside lesion
- Often several smaller satellite rings develop
- Rash or lesion may be itchy and irritating
- Rash usually disappears after a few weeks
- Some symptoms slowly subside within two to three years, depending on the build-up of antibodies
- Often symptoms recur with a vengeance with a new tick bite
- Phase One can last an average of three to six days; then the fever usually goes down
- Profuse perspiration can and frequently does occur
- Untreated or unidentified cases can progress to Phase Two and Phase Three
- Children often do not get this particular rash, but may have other rashes or hives. Some develop no rash at all.

Phase Two – Common symptoms

Within weeks to months later, but usually an average of five to ten days later these symptoms may appear:

Possible neurological problems

- Irritation to the covering of the brain (meningitis)
- Inflammation of the spinal cord and brain known as meningo-encephalitis. (Dr. James F. Balch in "Prescription for Nutritional Healing" mentions possible brain damage)
- Neuropathies of the cranium (cranial nerve disturbances such as Bell's palsy or Trigeminal neuralgia
- Inflammation of the nervous system, (Neuroborrelia)
- Facial paralysis
- Severe headaches
- Carpal tunnel (a peripheral neuropathy)
- Dizziness

Possible cardiac problems

- Inflamed heart muscle (Myocarditis).
- Inflamed heart lining (Pericarditis)
- Irregular heart (Arrhythmia, an electrical malfunction of the heart)
- Enlargement of the heart muscle.

Most of the following information came from a Lyme disease discussion on America Online, during which a Connecticut optometrist answered questions from participating Lyme disease patients. The doctor mentioned that a test for spirochetes in eye fluids should be but usually isn't being done. He suggested that patients insist on such a test (LUAT).

Common eye problems occurring with Lyme disease

- Moderate to severe floaters, caused by spirochetes in eye fluids
- After images
- Strobing, (strobe-like) vision
- Seeing bright disks when eyes are closed
- Peripheral movements (very common)
- Temporary loss of sight
- A few patients reported optic neuritis, a condition which frequently occurs in Multiple Sclerosis patients also
- Migraine headaches and other headaches accompanied by eye disturbance
- Black spots
- Blurred vision
- Sight is described as "foggy, steamy vision like looking through cellophane"
- Enlarged blind spots, evidently caused by optic neuritis
- Colored spots
- Light flashes
- Frequent occurrence of "pink eye"
- Retinal tugging (Physician commented, that this could be a factor if vitreous humor liquefies from spirochetes)
- Blepharospasms (twitching, sudden closure of eye lids)

Possible severe complications in Phase Two as reported in "Diseases", Nurse's Reference Library

- Nephritis
- Bronchitis
- Pneumonia
- Endocarditis
- Seizures
- Cranial nerve lesions
- Paralysis
- Coma
- Death may occur from Hyperpyrexia (very high fever)
- Massive bleeding
- Circulatory failure
- Splenic rupture
- Secondary infection

Approximately 15% of patients develop the complications of Phase Two within a time span of several weeks to several months following the tick bite.

Phase Three - common symptoms. These can occur within weeks to years after the tick bite

- Painful joint (arthralgia)
- Painful joints (arthritis)
- Almost all joints are painful (polyarthritis)
- Backaches
- Stiff neck
- Pain in knee joints
- In some cases a degenerative muscle disease develops.
- Severe disability can develop within several weeks up to two years after the acute phase infection. It is estimated that about 60% of patients experience this stage.

Untreated chronic cases may develop these symptoms:

Physical and neurological symptoms
- M.S type symptoms
- Meningitis
- Myelitis
- Measles
- Carpal tunnel syndrome
- Guillain Barre syndrome
- Bell's Palsy
- Trigeminal neuralgia
- TMJ (Temporal Mandibular joint) problems
- Parkinson's disease
- Alzheimer's
- Fibromyalgia type pain
- Muscle pain
- Chronic fatigue
- Shortness of breath
- Memory problems
- Brain inflammation
- Swelling of knee or other joints
- Enlarged spleen
- Enlarged lymph nodes
- Bursitis
- Epilepsy
- Paralysis
- Sudden deafness

Psychological symptoms
- Irritability
- Depression
- Mood swings

- Psychosis
- Dementia
- Confusion
- Prolonged crying spells

Current medical treatment
Are antibiotics effective?

If diagnosed immediately, antibiotics given during Phase One may stop symptoms and/or prevent complications in many patients, but in some individuals they are not effective.

Prophylactic treatment

There appears to be general agreement that prophylactic treatment is of "unproven value". A placebo (Penicillin) study revealed that the risk of allergy to the drug Penicillin is much greater than that of acquiring an infection. This study was published by United States health authorities.

When spirochetes attack already weakened tissue the effect can be deadly under these conditions:

- If the affected patient has diseased vital organs
- If the diagnosis is delayed and treatment is not promptly given
- Acute symptoms can continue for several weeks after the initial Phase One treatment, and some people will develop Phase Two and Phase Three complications in spite of antibiotic treatment.

Reference sources list these drugs of choice:

- Tetracycline
- Penicillin
- Erythromycin
- Cephalosporin

Patients and physicians on America Online discussed the following other drugs:

- Plaquenil - This is prescribed for Lupus in connection with Lyme disease. One patient discontinued drug because of severe stomach upsets. This drug does not kill spirochetes.
- Biaxin (oral) - Drug is very good penetrator of the CNS; breaks down the cell wall unlike Amoxicillin.
- Suprax is a third generation Cephalosporin; very potent against spirochetes. Suprax inhibits RND in cell membrane
- Combination of both works well for some, but other patients stated that they tried the Biaxin-Suprax combination, but had better results with Penicillin
- Another patient spoke about having success with higher doses of Amoxicillin, but not with Biaxin

Dr. Raf, during his AOL online presentation, gave this information about the LUAT test, which evidently is the only effective test, which can be used years after infection. The LUAT test does not look for antibodies to Lyme, but antigens in the urine. These are broken up spirochetes in the urine, usually seen after a Jarish Hersheimer reaction (massive die-off of spirochetes). The LUAT test is very effective in comparison to an only 8% positive result in blood testing. Evidently the patient is instructed to take antibiotics for a week to promote spirochete die-off and then urinate into a cup to provide a urine specimen on the day of testing. The LUAT test at the time of the AOL survey was done by IgxLab in Palo Alto, CA.

How does a patient know that he/she was bitten by a tick?

Many people have no idea that they were bitten, because the tick is no longer there. Only through a careful history about recent whereabouts and general symptoms can the doctor sometimes make the connection. Often such patients are treated for general symptoms.

Laboratory Diagnosis

- A lab test by itself cannot provide a solid diagnosis
- Blood testing for antibodies is done within three weeks after infection occurred
- Urine is tested for Borrelia burgdorferi bacteria (Please see "LUAT TEST"). The Borrelia burgdorferi spirochete can not be isolated by culture, and rarely do blood, joint fluids, skin scrapings and other clinical specimen lead to a positive identification thus complicating the situation.

Serologic Testing

Current serological tests are not sensitive enough to detect Lyme disease in the early stage. The author states that her own blood test, taken within a couple of days of the bite, resulted in a negative reading. Because of subsequent serious symptoms and insisting that the attending physician order a follow-up test about 6 months after the tick bite this new test showed a very high titer.

Current tests are not specific enough

It is common to see cross reactions with other spirochetes, such as those linked to "syphilis", "relapsing fever" and "leptospirosis". The Public Health Department admits, that both "false positive" and "false negative" serologic test results have been well documented. Standard testing can confirm only about 15% of a positive Lyme disease diagnosis within the first 20 days after the illness begins. The percentage increases to 27% when the test is performed within a three - six week period. And real evidence of antibodies is often not detectable until many months after the acute Phase One. Several reports state, that some patients never develop an antibody response.

"Nurse's Ref. Library" lists the following tests used for detecting spirochetes

- Wright's or Giemsa stain in blood smears during febrile period. Borrelia spirochetes are harder to detect in later relapses
- In severe infections, spirochetes are found in urine and CSF
- White blood cell count up 25,000, increased lymphocytes and ESR
- The WB may be normal
- Borrelia may cause a false test result for syphilis
- Standard tests: ELISA, Western Blot antibody test rate of false positives is 10%
- Rate of false negatives is 30%
- Some patients never develop antibodies to Borrelia Burgdorferi Bb
- DNA and Spinal = odds of positive are slim

The FDA approved a new blood test "PreVue" for Lyme disease in 1999. The reader is advised to ask their physician for further information.

Chapter III
What is a spirochete?

Borrelia spirochetes, responsible for Lyme disease can be seen under a microscope as small, flexible filaments, with 3-5 large wavy spirals, axis filament and periplast membrane.

Treponema spirochetes, responsible for syphilis have very tight close coils and banding, rotating movements, axis filament, but no crista.

Sometimes *Borrelia spirochetes* are mistaken for syphilis. Because of cross reactions with other spirochetes, some patients have been misdiagnosed with syphilis, when in reality they have Lyme disease.

What should you do, if you suspect a tick bite?

- If possible, remove the specimen, put it into a small container, add some rubbing alcohol and save.
- Call your local health department and ask for further instructions. You may be asked, to immediately contact

your physician, who should keep careful records of your symptoms and report back to the health department.

- You or your physician may be instructed to send the specimen to a designated lab. In the state of Washington, the state Public Health Lab performs only tests in cases with advanced symptoms and has discontinued "routine Lyme testing". Reader is advised to recheck this information for accuracy.
- Some private labs perform Lyme serology tests, and both commercial kits and services are now available.

It is important for the patient or health care provider to forward the tick specimen to a State lab with the following information:

- When collected
- Where collected
- Source or animal host, such as a dog, cat, deer, etc.
- Patient's name, address and phone number

Survey of symptoms listed by 50 patients compiled by the author from the Lyme Message Board, America Online

General pain

- Rib pain
- Pressure pain
- Muscle pain
- Head pain
- Shooting pains into feet
- Shooting pains into knees
- Tightness of tissue over knee cap
- Ear pain
- Severe shoulder and arm pain after anti-biotic treatment
- Sore knee joints
- Painful knots on bones (possible lymph congestion)
- Fibromyalgia linked to Lyme disease
- Pain swallowing
- Extreme sore spot inside throat on level with Adams apple.
- Dry eyes, dry mouth and pain inside mouth

Neurological and/or mental symptoms

- Fog-like state
- Spaced-out feeling
- Loss of feeling in upper lip
- Crawling sensations under skin
- Lesions found. First M.S. was suspected, but in this case the M.S. test was negative
- Feeling of "Saran Wrap" on face
- Feeling of paralysis left/or right eye muscles and nostril
- Numbness in outer leg
- M.S. - like neuroborreliosis symptoms
- Bell's palsy
- A.L.S. (Lou Gehrig's) - like symptoms

Sensory organ complaints

- Buzzing, ringing in ears
- Vertigo
- Spinning feeling
- Loss of sight in one eye
- Double vision
- Temporary vision loss in one eye
- Feeling of paralysis of skin surrounding the eye
- Heaviness of eye lid
- Feeling of pressure on eye lid
- Sjoegren's syndrome - like symptoms (dry eyes and mouth)

Cardiac/Circulation complaints

- Palpitations
- Shortness of breath
- General soreness in chest over the heart area

Immune system

- Swollen lymph nodes on neck

- Swollen salivary glands (parotid) with ear pain
- T-Cells affected
- Flu-like symptoms
- Erratic fever
- Bulls eye rash (typical for Lyme disease)
- Swollen glands

Miscellaneous symptoms

- Alopecia universalis (this could also be caused by medications)
- Feeling of hangover
- Severe allergies (could be caused by Candida yeast overgrowth, which is caused by frequent use of antibiotics).
- Epstein Barr- like symptoms, which in this case later were diagnosed as Lyme disease.
- Fatigue
- Insomnia
- Nervousness

Prescriptions discussed by patients during AOL survey

- Bicillin (patient saw no results)
- Bocephin 2 mg in IV
- Gammaglobula (spelling?)
- Claforan
- Doxycycline
- Vancomyacin
- Zovira for EBV and Doxycycline for Lyme
- IV Cephal
- Zithromax
- Xythromax Biaxin
- Amoxicillin
- Biaxin
- Suprax

Many patients reported many months and even years of antibiotic treatments. Other patients reported no improvements in spite of long-term antibiotic treatments. Some said that medication administered by IV was always more effective than oral therapy. One patient stated that prescribed "steroids" destroyed the central vision in one eye.

Medical treatment for Lyme disease as listed in various nursing journals 1983 - 2000

(Reader, note that treatment in 2003 may be different)

Oral tetracycline preferably by IV. If patient is allergic to this drug, then penicillin G is used. CAUTION LISTED: Neither drug should be given at the height of a severe febrile attack, because it causes a *"Jarish Hersheimer" reaction*. Please, read description below.

Jarish-Hersheimer symptoms:

- Rigors
- Malaise
- Leucopenia
- Flushing
- Fever
- Tachycardia
- Rising respiration
- Hypotension

The reaction is caused by the toxic by-products from massive spirochete destruction, which can mimic a septic shock and may prove fatal. Anti-microbial therapy must be delayed until the fever subsides. Until then: electrolyte fluids are supplied through IV.

- If tetracycline or penicillin do not work Chloramphenicol is used with caution
- CBC monitoring is needed

Many Lyme disease patients remain actively infected despite prolonged antibiotic treatment (Ref. Pat Coyle's

Study on Chronic Relapsing Neuroborreliosis, published by Stony Brook University) and information gained by speaking with Lyme disease patients about their treatment.

Complications with antibiotic treatment

Antibiotics can depress antibodies, and thereby interfere with the accuracy of tests. Antibiotics, especially if given repeatedly, can also cause very severe yeast-fungus overgrowth. If this problem (Candida Albicans) is not corrected, the patient could not only develop multiple allergies and sensitivities, but chronic fungal infections could cause serious, even life-threatening problems in lung and other internal tissues.

Very Important

What to watch for, if patient is sent home with medical antibiotics for treatment: Patient must be watched closely for any signs such as flushing, very low blood pressure and irregular heart beat. These symptoms must immediately be reported to the physician. Antibiotics cause massive die-off of spirochete bacteria. The resulting symptoms are known as a "Jarish-Hersheimer reaction" (see previous remarks). During the febrile period body temperature should be taken every two to four hours, vital signs must be recorded and level of consciousness observed. Caregiver must be watchful for signs of neurological disturbances such as
- Possible seizure activity
- Level of consciousness
- Tepid baths must be used to reduce high fever
Non-medical therapy used by some of the survey patients participating in Lyme Board discussion
- B12 shots which helped nerve pain
- Multi-Vitamins, extra fish liver oil, Coenzyme Q10 and B6. Patient felt better in general

- One patient reported that Rocephin plus B12 shots made him feel better
- Several patients reported that they were using multi-vitamin supplements plus extra vitamins C, B and E
- Others reported the use of many different vitamins, minerals and anti-oxidants
- Colloidal silver was used as a natural antibiotic
- Herbal product specific for fungal problems were used
- Tissue salts (also called cell salts). These are available as sublingual tablets in all health food stores.

Chapter IV
Discussion of Holistic Therapy Options for Lyme disease

Silver in colloidal form only (avoid other silver preparations) appears to be the most effective natural antibiotic available to Lyme disease patients and can be used safely without any side effects

Natural therapy options for coughs, sore throats and chills

- Colloidal silver (#1 choice)
- Vitamin C dosages, 5- 10 grams daily in divided dosages
- Zinc, 30-50 mg chewable lozenges or tablets
- Slippery Elm tablets to soothe irritated throat tissue
- Yerba Santa tea
- Ginger tincture
- Linden tree blossoms tea to promote perspiration

Natural therapy options to fight parasitic and other infections caused by Lyme disease

- Colloidal silver (#1)
- Vitamin C in high dosages, most effective when administered through an IV; otherwise as Ester C plus Bioflavonoids

- Kelp, tea or tablets
- Goldenrod tea
- Burdock. tea
- Milk thistle, tincture
- Yellow Dock tea
- Nettle tea
- Sarsaparillas tea
- Dandelion, tea from root and leaves
- Black Walnut, tincture
- Gentian, tincture
- Garlic, raw cloves, or as tablets
- Alfalfa, tea or tablets

Encephalitis in Lyme disease

- Horseradish is effective against tick-born encephalitis virus (ref. H. Kroeger Herbals)

Natural antibiotics for Lyme disease

- Colloidal silver (#1)
- Vitamin C in very high dosages, preferably through an I.V. in emergency cases; otherwise Ester C plus Bioflavonoids
- Garlic, raw cloves or tablets
- Raw unfiltered honey
- Echinacea, tincture
- Goldenseal, tincture
- Milk Thistle, tincture
- Red Clover tea
- Suma tea

Natural anti-bacterial substances and herbs helpful in Lyme disease

- Colloidal silver (#1)
- Vitamin C in high dosages; or Ester C
- Ginger, tincture (has antibacterial and probiotic action)

- Schizandra
- Gentian tea or tincture
- Burdock, tea
- Black Walnut, tincture
- Yerba Santa, tea
- Astragulus
- Echinacea, tincture
- Garlic, raw cloves, or in tablet form
- Goldenrod, tea
- Horseradish, which contains hydrogen peroxidase

Natural antioxidants to assist the immune system

- Vitamin C in mega-doses is a natural antihistamine, which kills bacteria and viri
- SOD (Super Oxide Dismutase); powerful antioxidant
- Vitamin E d-alpha and mixed tocopherols
- Vitamin A fish liver oil
- Beta carotenes and all other carotoids; found in red and green and yellow vegetables and fruit
- Zinc gluconate or picolinate
- B6 (Pyridoxine)
- Multi-enzyme combinations, which must include antioxidant enzyme Catalase
- Pycnogenol (Pine bark extract)
- Bromelain; anti-inflammatory; anti-oxidant
- Bilberry tincture
- Blue Elderberry tincture or juice
- Blackberry juice and fruit
- Black currant juice or extract
- Strawberries; fresh, frozen or juice
- Blueberries; fresh, frozen or juice

C a u t i o n ... The use of high potency anti-oxidants can produce a large die-off of spirochetes. Patient should remain calm, quiet, drink lots of fluids; eat a light diet, until flu-like feelings have passed. Please review Jarish-Hersheimer symptoms.

Natural helpful anti-inflammatory substances

- Colloidal silver
- Ginger
- Bromelain
- Tissue salt #4 Ferr. Phos.

Nausea

- Ginger, tincture
- Tissue salt #10 Nat. Phos.

Specific natural therapy options with homeopathic tissue salts

- For *fever*: Ferr. Phos. Tissue salt #4
- For *convalescence*: Ferr. Phos. #4 plus Calc. Phos. #2
- For *acute inflammatory pain*: Ferr. Phos. #4
- *Neuralgia pains*: Mag. Phos. #8
- *Inflammation*: Ferr. Phos. #4
- *Nausea*: Nat. Phos. #10

How to use specific vitamins, minerals and trace elements to fight Lyme disease

Vitamin C

To effectively fight any infection, including Lyme disease, vitamin C can be taken in daily dosages starting at 6,000 mg and higher. This nutrient works best when taken in divided small dosages throughout the day. Vitamin C is highly effective against bacteria and viri. Its antioxidant action protects the immune system against all kinds of toxins, including many toxic metals. Vitamin C helps to chelate toxic substances out of the body. Ester C products have a neutral ph and therefore do not cause irritation to the stomach. They also remain longer in the body and are more potent than regular vitamin C. In an acute health crisis, giving vitamin C by I.V. could be a life saver. Hopefully the reader can find a medical physician willing to prescribe such treatment.

Additional vitamin C information

Even before Linus Pauling became famous for his vitamin C research, Irvin Stone published his wonderful book about Vitamin C and its many protective functions. Vitamin C is known to enhance the effectiveness of antibiotics and aspirin. Vitamin C along with DMG (Dimethylglycine) has bacteriostatic action, which means that it stops the bacteria from growing. Vitamin C also has bactericidal properties, which means that this nutrient is a highly effective antiseptic. Irvin Stone listed vitamin C's bacteriostatic and bactericidal effectiveness against the following bacteria:
•   Staph. aureus (pus)

- B coli -
- B sublitis
- B diphtheria
- Strep hemolyticus and whooping cough
- Tuberculosis
- Leprosy

Vitamin A

The "emulsified form of vitamin A" allow us to take fairly high amounts of this nutrient. Vitamin A is a highly protective antioxidant and strengthens the immune system. Emulsified A is available in capsules of 25,000 IU. - 50,000 IU daily. It protects and strengthens the immune system.

Vitamin E

Vitamin E is most effective in the d-alpha form for circulatory problems, while the mixed tocopherol form is recommended for antioxidant purposes and detoxifying action in the liver. Recommended daily dosages: 400 IU, but not to exceed 1,600 IU/day. CAUTION: W. Shute, M.D., Canadian cardiologist and famous vitamin E researcher, cautioned in his book "The complete and updated vitamin E book" about the use of mega- doses of vitamin E by patients with a history of chronic rheumatic fever and those with high blood pressure. Such patients are strongly advised to follow Dr. Shute's recommendations regarding carefully tailored dosages of vitamin E. Please, read his book for specific instructions.

Multi-vitamin and multi-mineral supplements which include trace elements

Any patient under great physical, emotional or mental stress has greater nutritional needs than a healthy person. The average US diet is nutritionally so inadequate, that the majority of Americans already have substantial nutritional deficiencies. A person ill with the tick-transmitted Lyme disease is therefore encouraged, to immediately begin a program of optimum nutrition. This program must include a potent vitamin and mineral supplement.

DMG (Dimethylglycine), formerly known as B15

Russian research has provided extensive and important scientific data, that DMG has bacteriostatic action and is extremely effective for both branches of the immune system. It also has a very beneficial effect on peripheral circulation and is used as an important tool for the prevention of leg ulceration, peripheral blood vessel spasms, minor and major strokes.

Coenzyme Q10

This cellular nutrient can help any patient with chronic advanced disease. In order to achieve best results for the seriously ill patient, dosages must be at least 100 mg 3-4 times daily. This nutrient is very important to both the acutely ill and/or chronic patient. And anyone suffering from chronic Lyme disease has to have some hope to deal with their illness. CoEnzymeQ10 is available without prescription in all health food stores in potencies ranging from 10 to 30 mg for minimum maintenance, up to 100 mg for acute, advanced and chronic disease. Advanced cancer patients have reported great success with dosages of four daily doses of 100 mg each. Coenzyme Q10 is also available in liquid form, which can be sprayed under the tongue for immediate assimilation

Other natural substances which are helpful in Lyme disease

Chlorophyll

All plants contain chlorophyll. Chlorophyll plays a very important role in the detoxification process. Fortunately the patient does not have to eat six pounds of broccoli or pounds of spinach leaves. Pleasant tasting chlorophyll green drinks are available in all health food stores and can be used on a daily basis. Chlorophyll is also available in tablet form or powder form in individual foil packets. This product is easy to use and very effective in detoxifying the bloodstream of impurities.

Alfalfa

This plant is not only quite important as a detoxifying plant, but also provides important essential trace elements found deep in the soil. An Alfalfa plant can send roots down to a depth of over 30 feet. Alfalfa has been used by many arthritic patients for pain reduction, and is available in convenient tablet form. A minimum of twelve tablets daily is recommended for Lyme disease patients. Alfalfa works best, when taken in divided dosages throughout the day.

Kelp

Rich in essential trace elements, this sea vegetation product provides plenty of chlorophyll and trace elements including iodine for thyroid support. Both Alfalfa and Kelp are natural vitamin K sources, important for blood coagulation. Kelp also contains anti-oxidants such as selenium, germanium and silver.

Garlic

Most effective in its raw state (in comparison to garlic powders or garlic capsules or seasoning), raw garlic was used by the Roman armies to treat infected battle wounds. Today, science has accomplished many wonderful things with garlic. Important for the Lyme disease patient is the fact, that garlic is a powerful natural antibiotic. It should be used daily, to fight bacteria in the blood stream and intestinal tract. Odorless products are available, and should be used daily to help the body rid itself of toxic materials. Garlic also helps to destroy fungi in the blood stream, a valuable help for the patient with Candida Albicans.

- A combination of Nettle, Yerba Santa , Goldenrod , organic Tobacco and Monolaurin has been mentioned as a specific natural therapy for Lyme disease patients
- Several specific herbal combination tinctures for anti-fungal protection are available in all health food stores
- All berries contain important anti-oxidant substances and should be used freely.

Natural Pain Control for Lyme disease patients

MSM (Methylsulfonylmethane

This is a nutritional sulfur product. Sulfur is needed by the human body to make connective tissue, such as ligaments, tendons, muscles, cartilage etc.

Dosage for acute pain: One 400 mg tablet per 50 lbs body weight twice daily for 4 days, then reduce to 1 tablet for each 50 lbs. once daily.

Dosage for chronic pain: One tablet per 50 lbs. once daily, but increase again if pain becomes acute. These instructions are printed on the bottle and do not reflect specific recommendations by the author. Product is available without prescription in any health food store.

Pain control combination

Also very effective in fighting pain is this combination of vitamin C, calcium and manganese:
- 5,000 mg - 10,000 mg vitamin C daily
- 2,000 - 2,500 mg calcium, daily
- 50 mg manganese, daily

This effectively reduces back pain, a stiff neck, leg spasms and other muscular, tendon, or ligament discomfort When pain is gone, reduce calcium to 1,500 daily. Manganese then must be reduced to 15 mg daily. Vitamin C is effective against bacteria and viruses so that a high maintenance dose is of great importance to the Lyme disease patient. The author recommends, that at least 10,000 mg vitamin C in Ester form

daily in 5 divided dosages of 2,000 mg each should be tried
to reduce symptoms of fever and infection. The most effective
way to administer large dosages of vitamin C is through the
use of an IV. Vitamin C researcher Irvin Stone reports in
his book, that Polio, Meningitis, Hepatitis and Infectious
Mononucleosis are all diseases that could be stopped with
immediate high vitamin C administered through an IV.

A complete back-up mineral supplement is recommended
to avoid upsetting the mineral balance with single high
dosages of vitamin C.

For acute illness or infections vitamin C is most effective
in dosages exceeding 6,000 mg, since a healthy 140 lb. person
requires 5,000 mg daily just for maintenance. Anyone sick
with a disease or under high stress automatically requires
much higher amounts of vitamin C.

Other natural pain relief options

- Evening Primrose Oil
- Ginger
- Willow bark
- Perna Canaliculus is a source of Chondroitin Sulphate,
  which contains the much publicized "glycosamines". This
  substance brings much relief to patients with arthritis
  type pains. Today, many companies manufacture
  Glucosamine sulphate, Glucosamine chondroitin
  and MSM combination supplements. Recent articles
  name *Glucosamine sulphate* as the *most effective form of the
  glucosamines.*
- Bromelain, a digestive enzyme, has anti-inflammatory
  properties and is very effective by reducing pain.

Chapter V
How to use specific plants for landscaping to discourage tick infestations

Certain plants have pest-controlling properties and can be used in home gardens, to give a certain amount of protection against ticks.

Use these plants in the garden:

- Mint plants
- Parsley (herb)
- Dill (herb used to make Dill pickles)
- Onions, chives, leek and garlic
- Horseradish
- Chicory
- Lemon tree
- English Walnut tree
- Tobacco

Usually found in the forest and clearings the following protective plants could also be grown in gardens:

- St. John's Wort, a common weed usually found at roadsides
- Yarrow, usually found near pasture borders
- Wormwood

Found along roadways and the edge of fields, Chamomile

prefers gravelly soil and is usually found along gravel driveways:

Chamomile (easily transferred to garden)

Both European and American Chamomile can be used as a tick-repellent plant. Its dried flowers (tea) can also be used for upset stomachs and inflamed sinuses.

Final notes

The author wishes to emphasize again that when a tick bite occurs, medical treatment must be initiated at once to avoid serious complications. Once crisis care has been administered, natural methods can be used. Both colloidal silver and vitamin C are known to enhance the function of antibiotic medications. Only when medical crisis care is not available, should holistic alternative therapy be used as the only form of treatment. Colloidal silver acts as a natural antibiotic. Colloidal silver is the absolutely best germ fighter and has absolutely no side effects. It has been well documented, that while medical antibiotics are capable of killing only 5-7 different disease organisms colloidal silver is highly effective against as many as 650 different ones. Widely used as a natural antibiotic before the event of penicillin, colloidal silver is still used by many sick people. This product is available in all health food stores and through the internet. It is, in the author's opinion, the most important natural medicine a Lyme disease patient can safely take on a daily basis. But only the colloidal form of silver is safe for long-term treatment.

Best wishes for better health,
Hannelore Helbing-Sheafe, Ph.D.

Index

For additional reading these sources are recommended

"Herbal Insights", Summer 1996
"Prescription for Nutritional Healing", by James F. Balch, MD
"Diseases", Nurses Library 1983 - present
"Lyme Disease Message Board AOL"
"Gesundheitsvorsorge", Vienna Publication 1995
"Vitamin C", Irvin Stone
"Washington State Public Healthy Bulletin"
1995 until present
"The complete and updated vitamin E book", Wilfred Shute, M.D.

About the author

Hannelore Helbing-Sheafe was born and raised in Germany, came to this country in 1959, and married Harry P. Sheafe, a well-known chiropractic physician in the Pacific Northwest. Hannelore pursued her own career in the holistic field as a Master Reflexologist and Holistic Nutrition Counselor and Researcher while raising daughters Susanne, Karen and Christa. She published her first successful book "Reflexology, The Ultimate Health Connection" in 1987. This book was used as textbook for all workshops taught in the Northwest and classes taught at the prestigious Evergreen State College in the state of Washington. Her intense interest in the relationship between nutrition and disease during her 30- year practice benefited each of her patients. They not only received therapy for symptoms presented, but were given nutritional guidelines to address the cause of their problems.

She received her degree in nutrition in 1984 and chose the holistic therapy approach to skin diseases, hair and nail abnormalities for her dissertation. Out of the vast research material compiled emerged a new book "The Bare Facts", which explains underlying causes and discusses natural treatment options for most known skin diseases, hair and nail problems. Many other titles have followed since, including *"Connective Tissue Diseases and Holistic Therapy Options"*, *"The Bare Facts"*, *an encyclopedia of holistic therapy options for common skin diseases and nail and hair abnormalities"* and *"Reflexology, The Ultimate Health Connection"*, *a home-study course for beginners and advanced students.* A new book *"Nature's Pharmacy"* is *planned for publication in 2003. This book is an important guide to symptoms, known nutrient deficiencies linked to these symptoms, lists all vitamins, minerals and trace elements and their function in the human body, and – most importantly – provides highly detailed lists of food sources in which the deficient nutrients can be found.* The reader therefore can quickly find important nutritional information specific to a health problem and focus on the foods, which help to normalize the condition.